Recognizing and Dealing Allergy

How to Completely Cure Allergies Using Natural Remedies

By: Cindy Best

9781681279640

Publishers Notes

Disclaimer – Speedy Publishing LLC

This publication is intended to provide helpful and informative material. It is not intended to diagnose, treat, cure, or prevent any health problem or condition, nor is intended to replace the advice of a physician. No action should be taken solely on the contents of this book. Always consult your physician or qualified health-care professional on any matters regarding your health and before adopting any suggestions in this book or drawing inferences from it.

The author and publisher specifically disclaim all responsibility for any liability, loss or risk, personal or otherwise, which is incurred as a consequence, directly or indirectly, from the use or application of any contents of this book.

Any and all product names referenced within this book are the trademarks of their respective owners. None of these owners have sponsored, authorized, endorsed, or approved this book.

Always read all information provided by the manufacturers' product labels before using their products. The author and publisher are not responsible for claims made by manufacturers.

This book was originally printed before 2015. This is an adapted reprint by Speedy Publishing LLC with newly updated content designed to help readers with much more accurate and timely information and data.

Speedy Publishing LLC

40 E Main Street, Newark, Delaware, 19711

Contact Us: 1-888-248-4521

Website: http://www.speedypublishing.co

REPRINTED Paperback Edition: 9781681279640

Manufactured in the United States of America

Dedication

This book is dedicated to my precious daughter Stacy. We love you.

Table of Contents

Chapter 1- All You Need To Know About Allergy

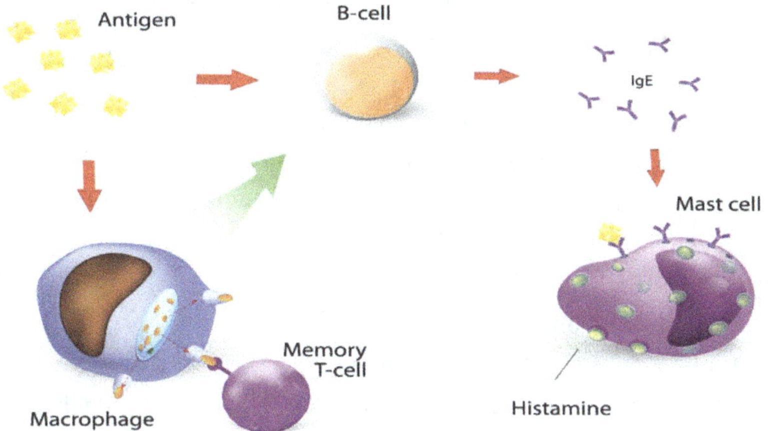

Today about 60 million people have some kind of allergy to one thing or another. It could be from the food you eat, or maybe the soap that you use, to the pollen in the air. There are so many of them that you do not know what to look for.

What are allergies?

Allergies are something that you get from an antibody called Immunoglobulin.

Antibodies are very important to us, since it helps to fight off any parasites, uniformly it does fight off the allergies since IgE or Immunoglobulin E affects the cells and tissues, causing damage.

What are the most common allergies that people get?

The most common allergies that people get are asthma, hay fever, allergic eye, emphysema, and hives. These are the most common ones you see today. There are outdoors allergies as well as in sides one. Rhinitis and sinusitis are common also.

One of the most common allergies that you may get is hay fever it is from the pollen in the air. Hay fever however is a seasonal allergic condition. Some of the insides allergies that you may see a lot are from dust mites and mold.

When you developed allergies, it causes your nose to swell, making it hard for one to breathe. This will cause the tissue inside your nose swells from inflammatory attacks. The white blood cells and mast cells are affected, which sets in inflammation.

There are little things that you breathe in called allergens. Once you inhale these, they can set in your ears, nose, throat, or your sinus. The most common symptoms that come from allergies are runny nose, stuffy nose, sneezing, nasal itching, itchy eyes, and postnasal drip.

Allergies can also cause your bronchial tubes to get inflamed. This will narrow the passageway causing you problems breathing. This can also cause you to develop asthma as well.

What are allergens?

Allergens are in the air that you breathe, they are in what we ingest, they are touching our skin, and they are everywhere that you can think of. What are allergens?

A substance that is foreign to the body's immunity system causes an allergic reaction. In some case mold and pollen cause such reactions.

Having allergies can make a person's life very miserable. Over 50 million Americans have been diagnosed with nasal allergies. There are many different ways to treat allergy symptoms using prescribed and over-the-counter drugs, yet because of many issues people still suffer. Consult with your doctor before starting any self-treatments, such as over – the - counter.

How do allergies occur?

Pollen and Mold are the two main causes for allergies in the outside air. Both natural air floaters are blowing around all around us polluting the air. Pollen comes from the grass, trees and weeds and mold comes from the leaves lying on the ground and rotting wood. Mold builds up in homes, especially around damp areas.

Our bodies produce two chemicals called histamine and leukotriens that cause the allergy symptoms. Most allergy medicines will block the chemicals that are causing the symptoms.

Symptoms of allergies are:

Runny eyes

Sneezing

Coughing

Stuffy nose

Keeping an ongoing list of allergies or what triggers them will help you a lot. If you know what allergies, you have than you can try to avoid them. By avoiding things you know will trigger your allergies, you'll feel better.

Some people often have to see a specialist who can detect what allergies they might have. Talk to your family physician and see how he feels if your treatments that you're currently doing doesn't seem to be helping.

By knowing exactly what allergies you have, it will be a lot easier to avoid being around them and they can be treated easier.

If you have upholstered furniture and carpets, try removing as much as possible. Carpets and upholstered furniture collect dust and pollens that float in the air. You can buy a special spray for the ones that you aren't able to get rid of. Cleaning for your carpets and furniture is very important to keep the dust out of them.

Check your mattress on the beds and spray them too. Get you a mattress cover with a zipper on it to keep the dust off. It is a lot easier to take a damp cloth and dust over the mattress every couple of days that spraying all around it and cheaper too.

Using air-filtering techniques to help reduce the dust and pollen that are floating through the air in your home can help reduce allergic-based pollutions. Do some research on the Internet of one and check out the best one to fit your needs? Air filters come in all different brand names, sizes, styles and prices make things easier on you and your wallet.

Pets are another one for carrying dust mites. Keep them out of the bedrooms and off the furniture. Some people have been known to have to get rid of their pets because of their allergies.

Many ways are available to cut down the dust and pollen that go along with allergies, so research is a good way to help reduce allergies to be healthier. Learn more about the environment and how it affects you also.

CHAPTER 2- COMMON TYPES OF ALLERGIES

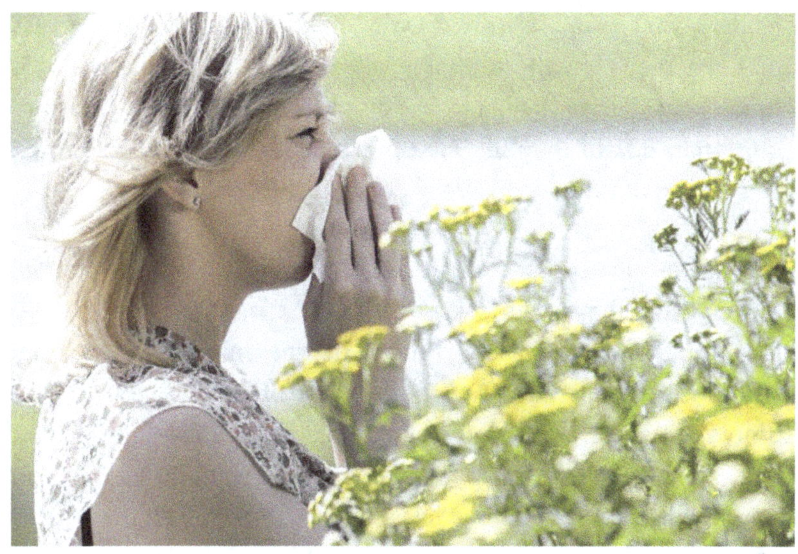

If you think you are prone to having allergic reactions to certain things, chances are, you may really be very sensitive to many types of allergens. The problem is, allergens can be anywhere and everywhere, and it doesn't help that our world has become teeming with noxious substances to add to other, more natural causes of allergies. Here are common types of allergies:

Dust Mites Allergy

Dust mites are in every ones house no matter how clean or dirty you keep your home. Dust mites cause allergies for many people. The mites can make it hard for you to breathe.

Dust or house mites are members of the spider family. They are little bugs that make you think that you have dust, but they really are little bugs that live and lay eggs. They can live up to 10 weeks; the last 5 weeks they lay eggs up to 60 to a 150 a day. They can live in your carpets, bedding, vacuum bags, and your furniture.

Recognizing and Dealing Allergy

Allergies have many different symptoms, so it is hard to say for sure. When you first start getting allergies you think it might your basic cold, so you take everything that you would as if you had a cold. You may even go to the doctors to get some medicine because what you were doing won't take care of it. Well, guess what the medicine the doctor gives you do not take care of it either. Now you are thinking what else it could be. So you return to your family doctor they set you up with an allergist. You get a test run and find out that you have allergies to dust mites.

There is not much you can do for dust mites. Dust mites appear all around your home, yet you cannot see them. You can be the cleanest person and there still might be dust mites in your home. They are so small they can hide anywhere. They can be up in the corners somewhere that you would think of. They love the vacuum bags. To get what relief you get, you might want to use a heap vacuum bag; this vacuum bag has a filter system in it so it will keep the dust mites.

Dust mites typically fed on furniture stuffing, pet hair and shredded skin cells from humans. It is possible to find relief from indoor and outdoor allergies.

Food Allergy

Nuts, peanuts, bananas, grapes, kiwi, eggs, milk, wheat, grains, soybeans, shellfish, fish, cherries, food additives, apricots, tomatoes, plums, avocados, melons, nectarines etc.

These allergens affect certain people. Bananas, cherries, grapes, nectarines, avocados, plums, tomatoes, and apricots affect many people, since these are allergic to latex. These are latex based bushes and trees which the fruits and veggies grow on.

Symptoms differ, depending on the food ate and the person's sensitivity to the produce. Diarrhea is common, followed by a series of other symptoms, such as nausea, and diarrhea. Rashes, itching, hives, and sometimes-asthmatic symptoms and eczema develop.

You can also experience some abdominal pain; this is normal as well as sometimes you could get an itchy mouth. This is also caused from food allergies. Swallowing can become hard for you as well as breathing can be a task for some people.

Food allergies can affect anyone at any age, from the first time a newborn drinks it could becomes allergic to the milk. If this happens, they will just change the milk to something else for example soy milk. However, for the most part of its children outgrow their allergies. Adults do not out grow them too often.

Mold Allergy

Mold is everywhere, including inside your home as well as outside. Many people are allergic to mold. Therefore, you need to try to prevent mold from entering your home as much as possible. Mold usually develops in damp areas.

There are various types of molds around and every kind can affect you in a negative way. Mold is also air born so that it can be hard to find in your home.

Mold can get in your nose and build up. You may not know until it attacks your respiratory and bronchial system.

Mold is normally found in many places where dampness is found. Such places like your shower stall, your basement, or a closet, even in the refrigerator in the fresh food drawer mold will hide. Mold can develop in your trashcan, or even in the laundry room.

Mold is outside. Mold grows on trees, even the ground. Sometimes, you see it growing in your home. Mold is all from the dampness outside. When it grows in your home its cause from too much moisture, so you may want to watch how damp it gets in your home to help count down the growth of the mold.

If you had allergies, I believe that you would know, but in some cases, you would not. Here are some things that you might want to look for. These are only the common symptoms that are associated with mold.

Nasal stuffiness, eye irritation, wheezing, cold or the flu like symptoms, could be a rash, fever, shortness of breath, fatigue, sometime even lung infection. Most of the time, these symptoms do not just go away it takes a long time to get rid of them. If this happened to you, you need to go see your family doctor before it gets worse.

Mold will also build up if the walls are moist. Some homes have moisture inside the walls. In this instance, black, orange, white and gray mold will often grow in the home. In this instance, you may need to hire a contractor or someone that specializes in home repair, etc to resolve the problem.

Physical Allergy

Physical allergies is commonly referred to for its name because if differs from most allergies. This condition is marked by reactions to physical stimulus that triggers the immune system.

Emotional stress, heat, cold air, sunlight, sweating, exercise, minor injuries, vibrations and similar responses are all responsible for physical allergies. The theory of the cause is that the protein changes in the skin and the immune system attacks it thinking it is a foreign object.

Some people are sensitive to the cold because of the abnormal protein in their blood indicating a serious condition such as cancer and chronic infections. People who are sensitive to cold will sometimes develop hives, asthma, nasal stuffiness, and swollen tissues under the skin.

Cholinergic urticaria is a condition resulting in itchy hives with redness around them. It is usually triggered by sensitivity to heat and any activity that causes sweating.

Studies are underway to find causes of these types of allergies. Some experts think that mistaking proteins is behind the problem. Certain drugs like cosmetics, creams and lotions along with the sunlight could be a link to the physical allergy.

When diagnosing what physical allergy reaction you have it is very important to monitor when the hives appear and what brought them on. The more information you doctor has the better is it to prevent you from going through a serious of test.

If you should break out in hives from being outside in the cold, tell this to your doctor and he can test it by putting an ice cube on your skin for 4 minutes. After removing the ice he can than watch the hives appear. This will tell him how to treat this particular condition

Emotional stress is something we all have at one time or another, but not everyone will break out in hives from it. Try to relieve as much stress as possible by avoiding it or maybe learning the technique of Yoga. Tell your doctors what happens when you become emotionally stressed and he can give you medication to help slow the stress down. You can also avoid stressors to keep stress at bay.

You will notice hives come up on your skin with redness around it.

The hives will appear for instance under the armpits or behind the knees after exercising. If you notice hives is sure to take notice what you were doing at the time they seemed to appear and consult your physician.

Exercising and sweating causes asthma to flare up or hives to appear under the arms, behind the legs, on your face wherever you might me sweating at. Some people only have this reaction when exercising.

Asthma is worsened when you exercise because of the fast breathing that cools and dries the airways. Usually happens more in the cold and dry seasons, causing wheezing, difficult to breathe, chest feels tight, and bringing out into hives as well. Stress is the number one factor however that brings on hives.

Seasonal Allergy

Pollen often causes seasonal allergies, which ordinarily is named Rhinitis. Pollen comes from weed, grass, trees and plants. The "male genetic" materials produce pollen from these natural resources. Units that hold male genetics are known as grain and have two surrounding walls to protect the grain. The intent is the deepest region of the grain that has thinning, delicate components.

The external walls are the exine, which has a high-tolerance to damage and is often thick. Pollination occurs when "pollen grains" are transferred. The plants transfer pollen grains from anthers and to male counterparts or organs. The male then transfers to stigma, which are the female counterparts.

After transferring is completed, fertilization begins. The pollen must go airborne to cause allergy reactions.

Cindy Best

Pollen makes up cereals, grains, weeds, grass and so on. The pollen produces from these natural elements in nature. Cereal pollen usually causes fewer reactions than weeds. Since weeds typically release higher volumes of pollens into the air, it causes episodes of allergic reactions for people in all areas of the world. Pollen typically causes Rhinitis.

The common weeds that affect people causing allergy attacks include ragweed, buckhorn plantain, redroot pigweed, nettle, Western water hemps, sheep sorrel, thistle, lamp quarter and the burning bushes.

What areas pollen usually attacks include Northern America and the Western Hemispheres.

During early spring pollen usually hits around February and up to March. Pollen hits late spring around April and throughout June and July. During summer months, pollen hits around June and carries on to August.

Ragweed grows in the fall. Some areas are isolated from pollen during winter months, yet in some areas such as South parts of California, Florida and Texas, ragweed will grow in the wintry months.

In most instances, people are allergic to one type of pollen or the other, yet other pollen allergies can develop.

As you can see pollen is an outdoor, irritant that affects millions of people around the world. To control pollen you should learn what areas produce high-volumes of pollination and in what months. During this time, you want to stay free of the outdoor areas where pollen circulates into the air.

Chapter 3- Ways to Win the Battle Against Allergies Naturally

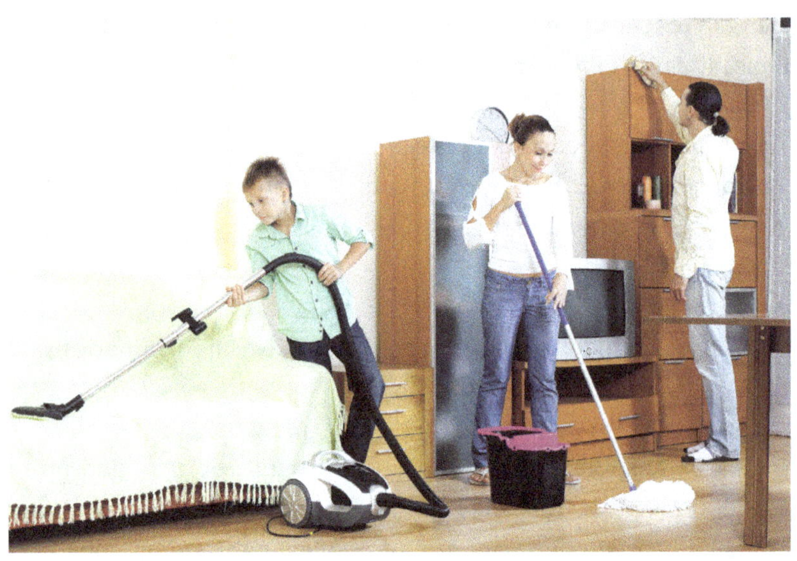

Millions of people are diagnosed every day with allergies. Allergies and asthma have the same symptoms. Both are treated sometimes with the same medication. Children are being born with allergies increasingly worldwide. Allergies and asthma have become a more serious disease as time goes and sometimes causing death.

Researchers have found that pollution is the main cause with all the mold and pollen in the air. Mold and Pollen affect the immune system in our bodies making us very sick. Researchers are trying to work to find resolves. Yet based on the fact that maybe sensitization of the immune system that is supposed to start doing its job really in life and been reduced due to modern hygiene. One of the big questions that remain, is could the drugs that are being used for treatment be part of the frequent recurrence.

There are treatments for allergy attacks. People can get a prescription from their doctor. The prescription is usually is an inhaler that you spray to help you breathe easier. Using the inhaler is only for short time use, not long term.

People have a tendency to overuse the inhaler even though their doctor warned them. Using the inhaler is a quick fix and people will use it because of the quickness and relief they get. If the inhaler is used as often, it can cause inflammation to set in the airways. Doctors no longer recommend that inhalers be used on a regular routine, they can cause more frequent and severity of attacks. Some people even turn to taking herbs, dietary supplements, and acupuncture as a short-term relief but don't last long.

Some doctors are now changing to different drugs that have anti-inflammatory in them. These drugs are very strong. The drugs could cause serious problems if used for long-term relief. People are known to gain weight; glaucoma sets in, hormonal changes and bone loss. Following your doctor's orders are very important with you, has allergies or asthma.

Thinking about the possibility that maybe your breathing patterns could be a cause, more of the attacks are a good thought. Remember how you panic whenever your breathing patterns change. In the past, do you recall any changes in your body that triggered your attacks?

We need figure out what is the real cause of allergy and asthma attacks. Consider the fact that every time you have an attack, it affects your breathing patterns and then you panic. Why did the pattern change?

Practicing and learning to control your breathing pattern is one way to help control our disorder with little effort. We are programmed from birth to breathe automatically, but it can be changed.

The breathing pattern can be changed with little effort depending on the function of your diaphragm. Your diaphragm is a strong muscle separating the heart and lungs from your stomach. Our brain sends a message to the diaphragm to activate it. Once the diaphragm receives this message, it flattens letting the lower ribs to swing out increasing the chest cavity. The lungs, then take over and create a partial vacuum pulling air into the lower lungs. We have to learn the process of when to inhale and exhale to let the diaphragm go back to receive another message.

Practice breathing and learn to control it. Changing your breathing might be the answer you've been looking for. Perhaps you need breathing lessons in allergy relief.

Breathing Lessons in Allergy Relief

Breathing patterns are very important if you have allergies. When a person can't breathe, they begin to panic and learning how to control our breathing is necessary for everyone. Changing our breathing patterns can be done with little effort. Some practice and learning techniques will help us to take control of breathing.

Breathing comes natural from birth and as we age sometimes, it needs to be changed to keep us healthy. In order to change our pattern we need to understand a little bit how the breathing technique works.

As we inhale our brain, sends a message to the diaphragm that is the muscle separating the heart and lungs from the stomach. When the message gets to the diaphragm, it activates it. It will flatten out, letting the lower ribs swing out so the chest cavity can increase. As the chest cavity, increases the lungs will pull air into the lower lungs.

When we exhale the lungs and muscles will go back to its normal size. After a pause, the process will start over again with the brain sending, it's message. The normal process of breathing is 14 times a minute more depending on how much the person needs it.

Breathing is controlled by the nervous system to run in its self-correcting mode. There are two branches of the self-correcting mode, one is "relaxation response" and the other is "fight response".

The relaxation response tells the system to slow the heart a breathing rate down. It works to keep the digestion and elimination going at the normal rate.

The fight response reacts to the functions that relate to emergencies and exercises. This response wakes and rouses our system to respond to the emergency by pumping adrenaline making our heart and breathing increases their rate. The increase will supply more oxygen to our bodies. If we are in real danger, the energy is used if not it could cause anxiety and hyperventilation.

With allergies or asthma, we tend to breathe faster not realizing it. Breathing at a faster rate will take more energy out of us, but letting us have more oxygen. At the same time, though when we breathe out we are losing too much carbon dioxide. If we lose too much carbon dioxide, it can be critical. The hemoglobin that carries the oxygen through our blood to the cells will become sticky not letting the oxygen through.

Learn to slow down your breathing rate to reduce your attacks. There are exercises that can be done to help you to breathe. Continue take all medications and consult your physician before starting to learn new breathing techniques.

Yoga exercises will teach you how to practice and learn new breathing techniques. You can join a Yoga group or buy CD's, videos and books about yoga. The materials to learn yoga can be bought at most videos and bookstores. Checking out the Internet is a great place to purchase these because there are some that can be purchased used.

It is a known fact that to practice new breathing techniques can help prevent attacks and help you to maintain a normal healthier life. Get started today and learn how to practice yoga for your own good health. By being healthier, you will have more energy to do the many things you've missed all these years.

Learning and practice is the next step for you and your health. The respiratory system requires care to help you find allergy relief.

Allergy Relief and Acupuncture

More and more people are known to have many different allergies every day. Allergies can be from food, cosmetics, radiation, sunlight, environment conditions, and allergens and just about anything you can imagine. Many health problems are related to allergic reactions and lower the immune system allowing other diseases to attack and weaken the body.

There is no known cure for allergy relief but ways to help prevent them or lessen the attacks. Knowing what to do for treatment and self-help will relieve you from a lot of pain and misery. Make sure you are suffering from allergies before taking action into your own hands by consulting a doctor. Your doctor can have test run to make sure he knows exactly what treatment is needed to relieve you from being so miserable.

Acupuncture may be the answer to your health problems by maintaining balance and harmony. After testing, to pinpoint the exact allergens that is giving you attacks. Acupuncture is a painless procedure, making the body strong where it was weak. Acupuncture reprograms the brain and nervous system. It does not react to the offending allergens.

Acupuncture is painless by using very tiny needles tapped in through a tub; so small that most people do not even realize they are inserted into the skin. This method is used for treating injuries and illnesses with drugs.

After acupuncture, you no longer need to avoid what was making you sick. This treatment rebalances your body energy when in contact with the offending allergens.

Allergy Relief Found in Yoga

Studies showed that yoga could reduce allergies over 60%. Yoga helps keep away allergies, asthma, and hay fever and so on.

Allergies can cause you to wake during the night, struggling to breathe, since the condition can cause suffocation. Allergies affect the chest; throat and breathing cause a person to feel stuffy. Some of the problems that emerge from allergies include sneezing, coughing, watery eyes, running nose, aching head, and so on.

Asthma and allergies affect millions of people each year. The condition wakes them up during the night hours, causing them to gag or gasp for air. Their breathing is often affected, which makes these people feel helpless.

Asthma alone can set up as pneumonia and can cause a person to grasp for air. Asthma affects the respiratory system, including the bronchial and pulmonary area. Asthma is a reversed disease that affects the lungs. This disease causes inflammation to attack the airway. The person will wheeze, struggle to breathe and so on.

Asthma causes flare-ups, coughing, swelling, muscle tightness, mucous buildup, and so on.

When a person is diagnosed with asthma, it causes swelling, which creates shallow breathing. The person will breathe heavily and swiftly gasping for air.

Some people are born with asthma, which goes away as they mature. In many instances, the condition turns to allergies. Some people, however continue life with asthmatic symptoms after birth and thereafter. Asthma may include mild symptoms, which develop into severe conditions. The condition is life threatening regardless. Asthma requires ongoing medical observation and treatment.

Allergies are affecting millions of people each day, yet to find relief individual studies must take place. We are all different, so we have to find what works best for us.

Studies show however that yoga is a healing agent. When we practice yoga, we practice natural breathing. Natural breathing helps us to take control of our respiratory system, complete body and mind. To practice yoga, however, you must have a will to take control of you. If you want, relief yoga is your answer. , You must continue visiting your doctor regularly to continue relief.

Using Herbs in Allergy Relief

Taking treatment with herbs is the all-natural way to stay healthy. Remember when taking herbs, even though they are considered safe, that some of them may counteract with your prescribed medications. So, be sure to read and learn about the herbs you are interested in taking to avoid problems. If you do not understand what you are reading and taking, consult with your doctor before starting anything new.

Some of the herbs that are being used today used for allergy treatment are Marshmallow root to help relieve mucous from the body. Burdock is used to clear the congestion in the respiratory system. To soothe, the throat and clear congestion, try using Mullein and to getting the antibiotic effect use Goldenseal Root it contains antibacterial and anti-fungal.

Eye Bright is a very effective natural herb to help the allergies by helping the congestion and hay fever that you might be experiencing. A natural antihistamine for allergies and fights infection use Capsicum. Stinging nettle is used to treat hay fever and another natural for the allergy treatments you're looking for.

Vitamin C and natural anti-histamine is found in Acerola Cherry. Rosemary is a good anti-inflammatory and strengthens the nervous system too. For reducing mucus and chest congestion, try White Pine.

Using herbs is just one way to help relieve allergy symptoms. Allergies can be deadly to a person if they are having chronic problems and do not get relief fast. When a person is having an allergy attack, they start to have a hard time breathing they can hyperventilate, and the oxygen level will go down. Remember herbs are not a cure they only help to relieve the symptoms. Consult a doctor if the symptoms do not seem to get better.

Cleaning for Allergy Relief

We have harmful chemicals and radicals in the air that affect our health. Recent studies showed that most homes have PBDE, which is a hazardous chemical. We also fight radiation, dust mites, mold, dust, mildew and other irritants daily. Sometimes it is difficult to find allergy relief, yet we must take action to save our health.

High-efficient air filters can help battle most microns and chemicals in the air. In addition, if we dust and vacuum our homes regularly, it can reduce irritants in the air. Particulate air filters can help you to avoid circulating dust back into the air.

You will find vacuums that do not use filters. This is ideal, since touching the filters after cleaning can cause allergy outbreaks. Always clean your hands after dusting, cleaning or touching anything that may have germs or bacteria around the area.

Clean Home Air for Allergy Relief

With the outside air being more polluted all the time, more people get allergies every day. When the air outside is polluted, it is 100 times worse inside. Most people spend more time inside where the air is worse than outside in fresh air.

The home environment is very important for people with allergies and the health of all your loved ones too. Get some cleaning done with an air filter today.

Poor air is not good for healthy people. It causes them to have headaches, fatigue, and irritation to the eyes, nose and throat. Your loved ones with allergic and respiratory problems need clean air to help them live a more normal life.

Air filters are used in your home to clean out the air pollution that is floating around. Using air filters will turn your air to crisp and clean air along with removing the bacteria, mole, virus and fungi. Your home will smell better and you will have less dusting to do.

Eliminating harmful odors such as paint smell, aerosol sprays and cleaning supplies are important and using a good air filter in the home can do this. Air filters break down the chemicals by breaking down the pollution eliminating many serious health issues.

There are many different kinds of air filters and sizes. You need to shop around to find the one to best fit the needs and air around you. Choosing an air filter is choosing the best one to fit best.

You might want to consider getting a small air filter for the bedrooms first. When you are sleeping, is when you need the cleanest air. The human respiratory system slows down when you are sleeping and can't handle the pollution as well as it can during the day. With a filter in your bedroom you will have a longer period to breathe in clean air, letting you wake up in the morning feeling more refreshed and less congested.

Air purifiers need to be running 24 hours a day to do what is expected from them. If you don't have enough money to buy, only in the bedrooms it is very important that you moved it out to the living area during the day to clean that air. Air floats and the pollution will go from one room to the other so keeping the air clean at all times is important.

Thinking about why you are buying an air filter will help you decide on the best one to fit your needs. People buy them just to keep the air clean for the new baby room, to clean the mold from returning, for the pet odors or specific health reasons.

Once you know why you're buying an air purifier for your home than buying the best one will come easy. Air purifiers come in many different styles so choose one of the specific reasons you are buying.

Buying air purifiers are not always the solution for people with allergies. As winter leaves, we're glad to see warmer weather, but dreading the allergies that come with spring.

Contacting your doctor is the first thing you need to do and get prepared. Ask your doctor for all the new information he can give you for allergies, contact your health insurance and see if they have a health calendar with dates that the pollution is at its highest peak of the season.

Vinegar and Allergy Relief

Chemicals can affect us in many ways. Some cleaners we use have harmful chemicals that can kill us if inhaled, or digested. We need to learn how to clean our home to avoid irritants that cause allergies. To get started, we need to consider chemicals.

Vinegar is distilled. It's made of grains and acidity products that come from natural sources. Vinegar has a strong aroma that sways most people from using the product, yet if you were to clean your home with vinegar, the irritants will stay away also. They too hate the nasty aroma that comes from vinegar.

Most chemicals we use for cleaning have hasty elements that interrupt the respiratory system, bronchi and sinuses. If we are to find allergy relief, we must convert to a new way of living. This means we should only use natural products to clean our home.

Lysol is a common household cleaning product. Many people use this product, yet some people suffer severe headaches after spraying the chemicals. Lysol has an active ingredient known as dimethylbenzylammonium chloride, which is said to eliminate germs.

The chemicals in Lysol are far less hazardous than other chemicals according to experts. Yet, the chemicals when overexposed to are toxic. The toxics are linked to birth defects, cancers, and have been linked to allergy attacks.

One thing for sure, many household cleaning products contain toxic. Not anything toxic surely should be worth letting into our environment. Most of your air fresheners, soaps, bleaches, shampoos, antiperspirant, hair spray, cleansers, detergents, and paint thinners and so on are toxic.

Still, we have to clean our homes. Instead of using chemicals with harmful Toxics, take your cleaning journey to organic reserves.

Vinegar is great for removing stains. Vinegar will keep away irritants. You can also use natural products made by SFI products. Most of these products are safe to use. In fact, thousands of people have tried these products and have given good reports. Go online to check reviews before considering the product. The vendors enable you to make money from selling the products as well. For the most part, you want to think health, so consider what you need to find allergy relief.

Filters in vacuums should be considered also when searching for allergy relief. High-efficiency filters can reduce irritants from your home over 90%. Hepa manufactured by NASA is one of the best filters on the market. This product was intended for use in plants, yet it was approved by proper channels and is now used in homes, hospitals and so on.

Cleaning beds and furniture is important. If you want to keep, dust mites and dust at bay wash your bedding weekly in hot water. You may want to add vinegar to your wash to help fight dust mites and dust.

Studies show that furniture made of upholstery has higher potentials of causing dust and dust mites to stick. If possible, you may want to invest in foam-packed furniture.

Wood collects dust. Televisions and carpets collect dust also. It is wise to cleanse the areas frequently. Dust at least once each day. To clean wood tries using the oils instead of the sprays. Oils are healthier for breathing than sprays.

If you have pets in your home, keep in mind that most allergies emerge from pet dander. If you are not prepared to separate from your friend, then take more time to clean your home. If you clean your home each day, you can keep irritants at bay. Perhaps you can designate one area of your home for your pet only. Clean air in the home is the start to allergy relief.

Having allergies is no fun and helping you or your loved one to be able to live a more normal life is very important.

CHAPTER 4- 51 TIPS TO FIGHT ALLERGIES

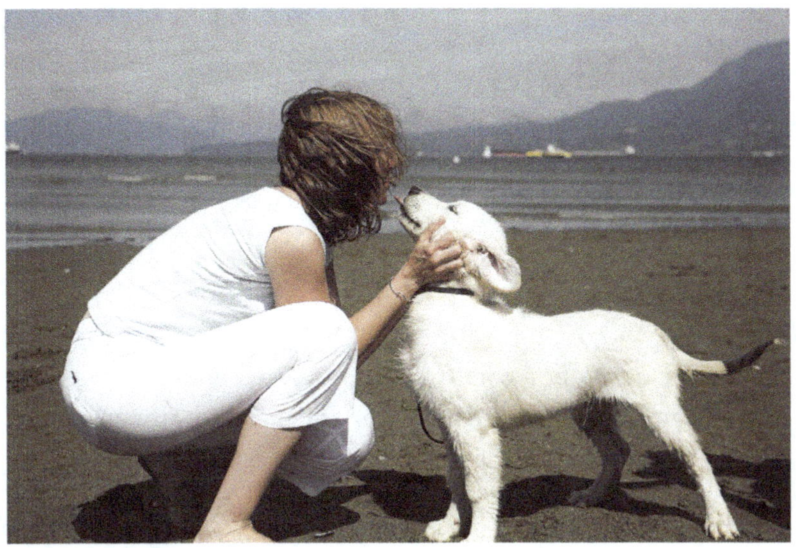

1. Avoid Early Ventures Outside

Avoid going outside between 5-10am. This is when the pollen count is the highest. If you have a pollen allergy, the safest times to go out are late afternoon and immediately after rain.

2. Check Pollen Count Daily

Pollen counts measure the amount of airborne allergens present in the air. They are reported as grains per cubic meter of air. Universities, medical centers and clinics provide these counts on a volunteer basis.

3. Turn off Your Swamp Cooler

People with severe pollen allergies may need to tough it out and keep that swamp cooler off during pollen season. Running swamp coolers can irritate allergy symptoms by dragging more pollen into the house.

4. Buy Local Honey

This may help to desensitize you against the pollens in your neighborhood. Many allergy sufferers claim eating local un-pasteurized honey has relieved their symptoms. They recommend you buy some local, unpasteurized honey and have a little of that every day.

5. Know Your Plants

Many people look at a colorful field of flowers and think it's filled with pollen. But those bright colors are there to attract insects, which carry the heavy pollen from plant to plant. The plants that aren't colorful are the ones that spread pollen...and allergies.

6. Wash Your Bedding

Your bedding needs to be washed in water at least 130° F to kill dust mites. Do this at least once a week. You can also use special laundry additive that kills dust mites.

7. Keep Indoor Humidity Low

Dust mites can't survive below 50% humidity (thrive at 75%-80%). It's a good idea to keep your home dry. Also, avoid humidifiers in bedrooms. If a sickness requires the use of a humidifier, you can get the same result with a steamy shower. Make sure you thoroughly clean the bathroom before and after.

8. Let Your Child Sleep With a Washable Stuffed Animal

If your child has allergies, let him sleep with a washable stuffed animal. This way, the dust mites can be regularly gotten rid of. If your child has a non-washable bedtime pal, you can put it in the freezer for 24 hours to kill dust mites.

9. Replace Old Mattresses

Depending on the age of your mattress, it can contain between 1 and 10 million dust mites. Unfortunately, unless you have a huge freezer, there's no way to get rid of them. The best solution is to toss that old mattress and start fresh with a new one.

10. Protect Your Bedding

It's a good idea to encase your bedding in an allergy-proof, dust mite proof enclosing.

• Pillows

• Box springs

• Mattresses

• Down Comforters

11. Use Dust Mite Powder

Sprinkle dust mite killing powder on carpet and upholstery regularly.

12. Don't Let Fluffy Into Your Bedroom

Keeping your pet out of your bedroom can at least cut your dander allergies down to half. Less pet dander in your bed may help you get a good night's sleep.

13. Bathe Your Pet Frequently

Long pet hair can trap dander, along with other allergy causing particles like pollen and dust. Bathing and gently scrubbing Fluffy frequently can reduce these allergens.

14. Groom Your Pet Frequently

Brushing your pet thoroughly and frequently can help reduce dander. Be sure and get a high quality brush that reaches down to the skin. Also, don't let pet brushes sit around. The hair and dander will wind up right back in the air, and in your nose.

15. Know Your Dogs

When shopping for a dog, keep in mind that there are certain dog breeds that have less dander than others. Among these are:

• Poodles

• Terriers

• Schnauzers

16. Minimize Indoor Plants

Though indoor plants are pleasing to the eye, they can make your allergies worse. They collect dust and can be a source of mold. If you can't bear to get rid of them, make sure you clean the leaves daily.

17. Thoroughly Clean

Make sure that any area that may collect mold is thoroughly cleaned. These areas include:

- Drain pans

- Shower curtains

- Damp basements

- Air conditioners

18. Avoid Line Drying

Don't hang clothes and bedding out to dry. Pollens and molds can collect on them. Using a dryer ensures that no mold will get on your bedding and clothing.

19. Use a Good Broom

There are all sorts of brooms out there. Choosing the right one can greatly affect the dust level in your home. Choose a broom that doesn't circulate dust back into the air.

20. Keep Indoor Shelves to a Minimum

50% of all dust in your home is on your shelves. Getting rid of the shelves you're not using can cut down on dust in your home. Also keep in mind that knickknacks on shelves can also collect a significant amount of dust. If you need those knickknacks, try getting closed door cabinets to display them.

21. Use Electrostatic ally Charged Dusting Cloths

Dusting with cloths or dusters can release 50% of the dust you're trying to clean back into the air. An electrostatic ally charged dusting cloth traps dust and doesn't let it back into the air.

22. Wear a Mask

Wearing a good HEPA (High Efficiency Particulate Arrestant) mask while you dust can really help with your dust allergies. Most of these block 95% of dust from getting into your lungs.

23. Don't Forget Hard-to-Reach Places

When dusting, remember to dust everything, including:

• Window treatments

• Windowsills

• Window frames

• Ceiling fans

• Light fixtures

• Storage units

24. B Complex

B vitamins are great for maintaining your nervous system. It can also act as an anti-oxidant and get rid of stuff stuck in your system that may be causing your allergies.

25. Vitamin C

Vitamin C is great for beefing up your immune system. It's just about the safest vitamin out there. A stronger immune system helps ward of allergies more efficiently.

26. Calcium

Not widely seen as an allergy fighter, calcium is usually seen as a source of strengthening bones. Certain studies, however, suggest

Cindy Best
that calcium can have an antihistaminic action. This means less sneezing for you.

27. Anti-oxidant Combination

Strengthen your allergy resistance with a good quality anti-oxidant. Combination includes the minerals zinc and selenium, and vitamins A, C, E, and beta-carotene. This combination has been known to have very good results in allergy sufferers.

28. Get Rid of Cockroaches

These nasty critters not only spread disease, but it's estimated that about 10 million people in the US are allergic to cockroach waste products. Cockroach sprays or traps aren't that expensive, and it will give you peace of mind to get them out of your home.

29. Avoid Ionizing Air Cleaners and Ozone Generators

Don't believe everything you hear. According to the EPA (Environmental Protection Agency), ionizing air cleaners and ozone generators are not only ineffective air cleaners, but they and can be very dangerous.

30. Use Allergy Medications Carefully

There are tons of over-the-counter medicines out there. Make sure you read the directions and use them carefully. Especially be careful with those that cause drowsiness. Be smart about driving and other things when you take them.

31. Wear a Face Mask

Face masks can really help people with bad allergies. Wear a mask while doing allergy-irritating projects, like:

• Mowing the lawn

- Cleaning a dusty attic

- Vacuuming

- Cleaning the bathroom

- Changing the bedding

- Grooming your pet

32. Avoid Alcohol

Alcohol can worsen nasal allergies. It stimulates mucus production, aggravating nasal congestion and runny nose. So think twice about medication.

33. Use Filters

Placing filters over heating and cooling vents can help alleviate allergies. Vent filters can trap airborne particles like dirt, lint, dust mites and hair. Filters aren't very expensive and can be found at any hardware store.

34. Choose New Carpet Carefully

If you're in the market for new carpet, it's important to remember that from an allergy sufferer's view, not all carpet is the same. New carpet can be a source of chemical emissions and irritants. Ask your carpet guy what chemicals were used on your carpet and give it time to air out. Serious allergy sufferers may want to consider hardwood floors.

35. Thoroughly Clean Down

Down comforters, pillows or feather beds can be hard to clean, but are also good at trapping dust and dirt. It may mean a trip to the dry cleaners, but the results are well worth it. You can also look for hypoallergenic down. This is specially made for allergy sufferers and will greatly reduce allergens.

36. Shower Before Bed

Showering and washing your hair before going to bed can greatly reduce your night-time allergies. During the day, you can get dust mites, pollen and even mold on your skin and hair. Showering at night will keep these things out of your bed.

37. Clean Your Floors

It's important to clean all floors in your home twice a week. This ensures that allergens are being disposed of. A good way to do this is to vacuum the area, then go over the floor with a wet rag or clean mop.

38. Avoid Smoke

This may sound like a no-brainer, but many people don't realize how smoking tobacco can actually make their allergies worse. Smoking weakens your immune system, making it easier to be effected by allergens. Also keep in mind that the air around people who smoke actually makes a great place for mold to grow.

39. Disinfect

A few times every month, clean all of your bathroom and kitchen surfaces with an industrial grade disinfectant (not just a spray disinfectant like Lysol). This will make sure that all of the allergy-causing germs are out of your home. This is also the best way to kill mold.

40. Clean Your Carpets

Make it a habit to have your carpets professionally cleaned each fall, after you close your windows for the winter. Do your homework, and ask your carpet cleaners if their service will get rid of mold, pet dander and dust mites.

41. Keep Your Windows Closed

A good rule for a serious allergy sufferer is to keep your windows in your house and car closed all year. Use the air conditioner instead. This makes sure those allergens outside won't blow into your car or home through your windows.

42. Drink Plenty of Water

A good tip for an allergy sufferer is to drink at least one gallon of water per day. This may seem like a lot, but it can actually help quite a bit. Along with flushing toxins out of your body, water also hydrates you. When your body is sufficiently hydrated, allergens don't stick as much and collect in your throat and lungs.

43. Exercise

Exercising daily will boost your immune system. Research shows that moderate exercise such as jogging, cycling and speed walking can boost the body's defenses against viruses, bacteria and allergies. Don't overdo it, though. Exercising too much can actually weaken your immune system.

44. Talk to Your Doctor

It's important to talk to your health care professional about your allergies. Whether it's your family doctor or an allergist, good communication is important to receive the best treatment for your allergies. Web MD suggests asking these questions:

• What substances are causing my allergies?

• What allergy symptoms should I be concerned about? When is it necessary to call the doctor?

• What allergy medications or other treatments are available? What are the benefits/side effects of each treatment?

• Will I need allergy shots?

• What guidelines should I follow if I'm prescribed allergy medication?

• Should I take medicine all the time or only when my allergy symptoms become worse?

• Should I stop exercising outside if I have allergies?

• What types of plants are better to put in my yard if I have allergies?

• How can I avoid or reduce exposure to certain allergens?

• What can I do around my house to reduce allergens?

• Should I avoid going outside during certain times of the year? What can I do to decrease allergy symptoms when I do have to go outside?

• How can I tell the difference between allergies and a cold or the flu?

• Will changing my diet to improve my symptoms?

• How often should I come in for follow-up appointments?

45. Use a Good Vacuum

Using a good vacuum is important. Your vacuum should have strong suction, adjustable brushes and high-efficiency filtration.

46. Take Care of Your Vacuum.

Experts recommend vacuuming floor coverings once a week; Pet areas; twice a week. Vacuuming furniture is just as important. This can put a lot of wear and tear on your vacuum. Make sure to change the disposable bag in your vacuum regularly (or clean the collector cup). Also check and watch out for worn belts.

47. Keep Bugs Out

Avoid attracting insects into the kitchen. These insects can make allergies worse. Here are a few things you can do:

• Get rid of all excess grease

• Keep food off of counters

• Seal cracks around cabinets

• Store food in tightly closed containers.

48. Use HEPA Filters

As mentioned before, HEPA stands for (High Efficiency Particulate Arrestors). A HEPA filter traps particles as tiny as .3 microns. To give you an idea what this means, Pollen ranges between 5-100 microns. Having a HEPA filter in your home will greatly reduce allergens.

49. Wash Your Hands

Yet another no-brainer, it's important to wash your hands and skin regularly. This will keep any pet dander, pollen or mold off your hands. This is extra important if you rub your eyes or mouth.

50. Use Dehumidifiers

If you live in a humid environment, you might want to invest in some dehumidifiers for your home. They're not very expensive, and can really help reduce dust mites and mold. If you already have a dehumidifier, here are some tips to remember for maintaining it:

• Change the filter once a year, so it will run at optimum performance.

• Clean the water container often to avoid mineral build up in the pan.

• Inspect the cooling coils for frost or ice build-up, as this can destroy the machine.

• Don't turn your dehumidifier off and then on again right away. Wait at least ten minutes to let the pressure in the system equalize.

• Don't set the humidistat higher than necessary or it will run constantly.

51. Do your own Research

There are constantly new ideas and tips for fighting allergies. Remember to do your own research. Use the Internet, newsletters, library, etc. You may find things that give you relief from your allergies that aren't mentioned here.

Chapter 5- Effective Herbs for Allergies

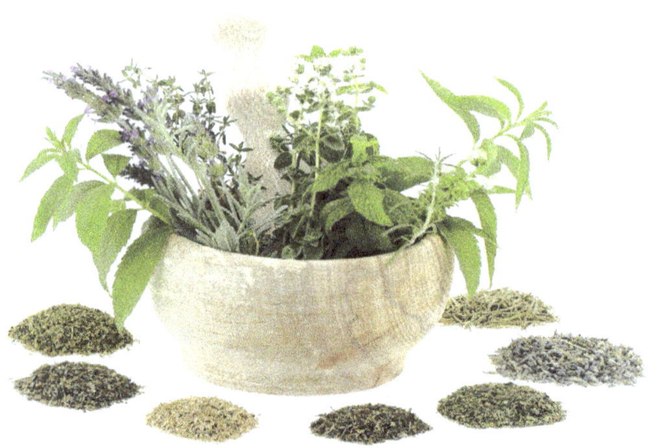

With the advances in today's medical technology, it seems new drugs and medications are coming onto the market daily. When it comes to allergy medications, it seems there is an over abundance of choices. However prescription drugs often have side effects that can sometimes seem worse than the allergies they are treating. However a recent trend has been for more people to look towards nature for help and many people find that helps using herbs for allergies with great success

Papaya - Although not actually an herb papaya contains an enzyme called papain that is commonly used to treat digestive problems. This enzyme also has shown positive results for allergy sufferers as well.

Vitamin C - Although mainly thought of as an immune booster vitamin C has very good antihistamine properties. And studies have shown a decrease in nasal congestion when combined with vitamin B.

Turmeric - Turmeric is an herb for allergies that is a main ingredient in curry powders and some hot mustard. It has shown to be a very good at reducing inflammation in asthma and allergy patients.

Quercetin - This is a very effective herb that can reduce the symptoms of your allergies after they have become uncomfortable due to its ability to reduce any swollen membranes in the nasal and sinus passages.

Cassia Seed - This herb has actually been proven to reduce temperatures in the body and provide relief for itchy and inflamed eyes. It has also been said to reduce the pain from headaches as well.

Rosemary - Rosemary stimulates your immune system, enhances circulation and improves your digestion. It also contains exactly the kind of anti-inflammatory compounds that you need to fight asthma. Add this to the fact that it contains polyphenols which are widely recognized to be amongst the most effective natural antiviral and antimicrobial compounds, and you can see that rosemary is a very powerful herb indeed which can play a vital role in your fight against asthma.

Oregano - It is believed that the antioxidant abilities of the natural chemicals in oregano are up to 20 times more powerful than those of any other herb. It also has strong microbial characteristics as well as being a rich source of many of the vitamins that you need in a balanced diet. Add this to the fact that it contains omega-3 fatty acids and you have another herb that you should include in your daily diet (it's great on pizzas and pasta in particular).

Dill - Dill has been yet another herb with acknowledged antioxidant qualities that also provides a significant source of calcium, thereby protecting against bone loss. It is also a rich source of trace minerals such as manganese, magnesium and iron, all of which you need as part of a healthy diet that you must consume in your natural battle against asthma.

Tarragon - Tarragon is a member of the dandelion and daisy family, an herb that is once again extremely rich in antioxidants as well as antibacterial and anti-inflammatory agents. Furthermore, it helps to strengthen your immune system and to protect your liver at the same time.

Motherwort - Motherwort is an herb that is highly effective for opening up the airways completely naturally, as well as having the ability to relax anyone who takes it so that stress and anxiety which can aggravate asthma are both lessened.

While not all herbs for allergies will work for everyone, they are definitely worth experimenting with because of the wow side effects they produce as well as being more affordable in most cases. But as with any treatment you decide to try always discuss it with your doctor.

ABOUT THE AUTHOR

Cindy Best is a Food Allergy blogger. As the mother of five young children, one of whom with severe food allergies, Cindy also spends much of her free time advocating for food allergy awareness and improving school nutrition. She volunteers and speaks on behalf of food allergy organizations. She lives in Southern California with her husband and five children.

www.ingramcontent.com/pod-product-compliance
Lightning Source LLC
Chambersburg PA
CBHW050706250726
48662CB00002B/873